HUNTINGTON'S DISEASE

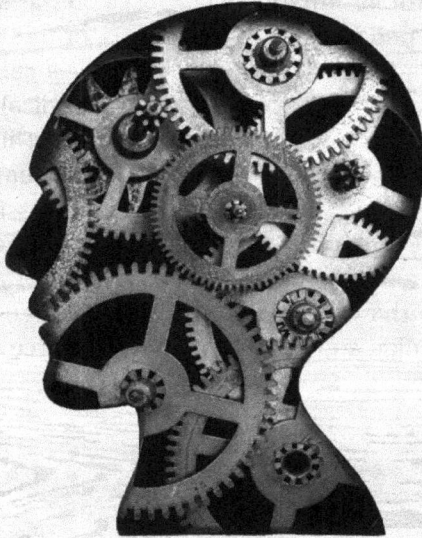

Activities for the Family Caregiver
HOW TO ENGAGE, HOW TO LIVE

Endorsed by

National Council of
Certified Dementia Practitioners

Scott Silknitter, Robert D. Brennan,
and Vanessa Emm

Disclaimer

This book is for informational purposes only and is not
intended as medical advice, a diagnosis, or treatment.
Always seek advice from a qualified physician about
medical concerns, and do not disregard medical advice
because of something you read in this book. This book
does not replace the need for diagnostic evaluation,
ongoing physician care, and professional assessment of
treatments. Every effort has been made to make this book
as complete and helpful as possible. It is important,
however, for this book to be used as a resource and idea-
generating guide and not as an ultimate source for a
plan of care.

ISBN 978-1-943285-19-8

Published by
R.O.S. Therapy Systems, L.L.C.
Greensboro, NC
888-352-9788
www.ROSTherapySystems.com

Introduction:
Activities for the Family
Caregiver—Huntington's Disease

This book is designed as a basic guide for family caregivers. The intent is to provide helpful information which includes leisure activities, activities of daily living, safety, and general caregiver information.

With the assistance of Robert D. Brennan, RN, NHA, MS, CDP, and Vanessa Emm, BA, ACC/EDU, AC-BC, CDP, who have been working in senior care for a combined 60 years, we have written this book full of How To's" and "Why's" to help you engage your loved one.

We hope you find it useful, and we encourage you to have other family members and caregivers of your loved one read this book in order to be consistent with approaches, verbal cues, physical assistance, and modifications that produce positive results.

From our family of caregivers to yours, please remember that you are not alone, and to never give up.

Scott Silknitter

Table of Contents

1. Huntington's Disease Overview   1

2. Personal Care, Activities,   15
   and Help You Bring In

3. First Pillar of Activities: 23
   Know Your Loved One—
   Information Gathering and Assessment

4. Second Pillar of Activities: 34
   Communicating and Motivating for Success

5. Third Pillar of Activities: 55
   Customary Routines and Preferences

6. Fourth Pillar of Activities: 61
   Planning and Executing Activities

7. Leisure Activity   65
   Categories, Types, Topics, and Tips

8. Activities of Daily Living   74
   Tips and Suggestions

9. Put Your Mask on First   98

Personal History Form   102

About the Authors   110

Family Members and Caregivers
that have read this book:

_____

_____

_____

_____

_____

_____

_____

_____

_____

_____

_____

_____

Chapter 1

Huntington's Disease Overview

Huntington's disease (HD) is a disease that causes the breakdown of nerves in the brain. It is hereditary and progressive. HD can affect all aspects of your loved one's life. Usually it causes cognitive, movement, or even psychiatric disorders with a wide variety of signs and symptoms. For the purpose of this book, we will focus on the cognitive and movement items related to leisure activities and activities of daily living. This disorder is caused by a single faulty gene responsible for a protein known as "huntingtin." Huntington's disease is a progressive brain disorder. The faulty gene is "dominant," meaning that anyone who inherits it from a parent will eventually develop the disease. This disease affects not only the loved one, but the entire family.

Symptoms will appear gradually but your loved one should be able to maintain their independence for years. To date, there is no cure or way to slow the changes that occur within the brain because of the disease. The clinical and social treatments focus on managing symptoms and working with remaining abilities. This book, as with all R.O.S. *Activities for the Family Caregiver* books, focuses on the social model of care and focuses on what your loved one can still do with their remaining abilities.

Regardless of how it is described, Huntington's disease is a struggle for everyone involved— your loved one, you as the caregiver, your family, and your friends.

Your loved one did not choose to have Huntington's disease. It was predetermined at birth. You did not choose to become a caregiver. Now that they have both happened, you must be prepared to work with, and adapt to, the changes occurring in your loved one.

Symptoms of Huntington's Disease

Symptoms usually develop between the ages of 30 and 50.

The average duration of the disease is 20 years, and the symptoms can vary significantly from person to person. There are no set patterns of development, and some of the symptoms may have a greater effect on one person than another.

With early onset Huntington's disease, different symptoms may occur at first, and progression is usually faster. An individual who has previously been healthy and agile gradually develops problems involving fidgeting, coordination issues, dexterity issues, and involuntary movement. Over time, chorea (involuntary jerking and writhing movements) may appear in the person's fingers, toes, face, head, neck, or torso. In some individuals, the movements may be very slow and take the form of dystonia (posturing or sustained involuntary muscle contractions).

Slow movement or bradykinesia (a general reduction of spontaneous movement) leads to impaired coordination and dexterity. Changes in intellect may precede or follow motor skill impairments by months or even years. The first signs of intellectual damage typically include an impaired ability to carry out a sequence of tasks, such as preparing a recipe, maintaining a changing work schedule, or overseeing family finances. Eventually a person's memory, recall, and learning are affected. Many other intellectual operations, such as language, spatial skills, and recognition processing, as well as the general fund of knowledge, may remain relatively well preserved. With time, however, your loved one's progressive intellectual decline may affect their judgment, analytic skills, and capacity for self-care.

Huntington's disease usually causes changes in the following areas:

- Movement (Motor)
- Cognition

- Behavior
- Psychiatric

Motor Symptoms

- Early signs may include clumsiness, loss of balance, and fidgeting.

- Chorea, the hallmark symptom with this disease, is uncontrolled movements of the arms, legs, head, face, and upper body.

- Muscle problems, medically known as dystonia, where the muscle and its tendons shorten, resulting in reduced flexibility.

- Impaired gait (a person's manner of walking, stepping, or running), posture and balance.

- Muscle rigidity is a state of continuous firm, tense muscles with marked resistance to passive movement.

- Difficulty with speech and swallowing.

Cognitive Symptoms

- Difficulty focusing on tasks.

  ○ Your loved one may have difficulty deciding what to eat, or they may have difficulty finding the ingredients needed if preparing a meal.

- Easily distracted away from a task at hand to another task or activity without appropriate follow-through.

  ○ Your loved one may start making a meal but may not finish.

  ○ Your loved one may eat a meal and may not clean up dishes, counters, pots, and pans, which is something they used to do.

- Perseveration, which exhibits as getting stuck on a thought, behavior, or action. For example:

  ○ Repetitive movements, e.g., stomping feet, raising arms, and shaking head back and forth.

- Repetitive verbalizations, e.g., repeating the same word(s) or phrase(s).

- Frustration, anger, or irritation in relation to one's thought process.

- Inability to finish/complete a thought— stuck on a word or phrase that has slipped away.

- Difficulty following other's conversations, movies, and TV shows.

- Slowness in thought process or finding words. For example:

We all have those moments when we say, "What is the word I'm thinking of? You know, it means _____." This type of dilemma may occur more frequently with your loved one which could lead to behaviors related to frustration. Allow time for your loved one to communicate with no sense of urgency or frustration. It may take several minutes for them to communicate a simple request. Make sure all caregivers know this.

- Difficulty learning new information.

- Long-term memory usually remains fairly intact while short-term memory is more difficult. For example:

  Memories of your loved one's childhood and early adulthood may be intact, and bits and pieces of those memories may be recounted, however, they can also be confused with reality. Your loved one may discuss something they used to do with their mother, father, or sibling but will display difficulty or no recollection of what they had for breakfast, if they paid a bill, what activities they did the day before, etc. Oftentimes these difficulties are displayed in waves or "good days" and "bad days." If this is happening often, it's a great opportunity to reminisce and discuss the memories that they do recall and want to share. Look through old photo albums, videos, etc.

Behaviors

- Lack of impulse control. For example:

  ○ Inappropriate language/cursing

  ○ Blurting out

  ○ Difficulty sitting and focusing on a task

  ○ Inappropriate sexual impulses

  These behaviors could also be displayed or masked as anxiety or anxiousness. They may occur during times of stress or confusion.

- Lack of awareness regarding behaviors they are exhibiting. For example:

  ○ Denial

  ○ Total unawareness of behaviors

  ○ No accountability for actions

- Unregulated emotions, mood swings, and anger. For example:

  ○ Overreaction to situations that aren't pleasing

  ○ Arguing frequently

- Noticeable highs and lows—feeling great/feeling sad

- Unwarranted anger toward loved ones

It's important as a caregiver to address each behavior and try to identify any triggers that contribute to the behavior or action. When do the majority of behaviors occur? What is happening before and after a behavior occurs? Once you are able to identify the main triggers, you can work on interventions and approaches to help alleviate and divert away from behaviors. This allows you to better assist your loved one through difficult times of the day. **For example:**

- Your loved one may overreact to everyday events when they did not before, e.g., not being able to find their shoes, lunch is late, or they do not like the outfit you have on.

- Your loved one may say cruel things or behave aggressively. Remember it is the disease process—try not to take things personally.

Psychiatric Symptoms

- Depression that has not resulted from receiving the diagnosis of Huntington's disease but seems to result from injury to the brain and changes in brain function related to the disease.

- Anxiety

- Insomnia

- Fatigue and loss of energy

- Thoughts of death, dying, or suicide

- Obsessive-compulsive disorders

- Mania (elevated mood, overactivity, inflated self-esteem)

- Bipolar disorder (alternating between depression and mania)

Stages of Huntington's Disease

As we all have unique personalities, each individual may exhibit different symptoms at different times/stages. The progression of the disease, however, can be divided roughly into three stages: Early Stage, Middle Stage, and Late Stage Huntington's disease.

Early Stage Huntington's Disease

- Subtle changes in coordination
- Some chorea (involuntary jerking and writhing movements)
- Depressed/irritable mood
- Less ability to work at the level they are accustomed to
- Less functional in regular activities
- Weight loss

Middle Stage Huntington's Disease

- Increase in movement disorders
- Diminished speech
- Difficulty swallowing
- Daily routines and activities become increasingly difficult, e.g., walking, picking up items, and setting the table
- Weight loss

Late Stage Huntington's Disease

- Choking becomes a major concern
- Chorea may be severe or may cease
- Can no longer walk
- Unable to speak
- Swallowing becomes more difficult
- Weight loss

However, it is important to remember:
Your loved one still, for the most part, does retain awareness of those around them and is still able to comprehend language.
It is important to maintain appropriate medical therapies to assist your loved one in:

- Medication management for movement and psychiatric disorders
- Physical therapy to keep strength
- Occupational therapy to help with activities of daily living
- Speech therapy for continuous evaluation of swallowing ability

No matter what stage Huntington's disease your loved one is in, they are still able to be engaged in an activity.

Chapter 2

Personal Care, Activities, and Help You Bring In

Having gained an understanding of the very basics of Huntington's disease, we now turn to you, your loved one, and others that may help in caregiving.

It is important that you recognize various personal attributes and abilities of your loved one and yourself. The better you know yourself, you can identify where you may need help. The better you know your loved one, who they are today, and who they were, the greater your opportunities for engagement and communication.

Huntington's disease may or may not affect your loved one's personality, but over time, it will affect and limit their ability for movement in addition to cognitive and psychiatric disorders. Behavior changes may also occur.

As the disease and symptoms progress, it is important to concentrate on what your loved one can do. Focus on and plan activities based on their remaining abilities using their preferences and likes as a guide to the topic of each activity. The more you know about your loved one, the more effective you can be as a caregiver.

Huntington's disease is an inherited disease caused by a defective gene. The Huntington's Disease Association notes that one in every 10,000 has the disease, and tens of thousands who have a parent with HD have a 50% or greater risk of inheriting the defective gene and developing the disease.

This book was made for the families and informal caregivers who care for their loved ones with Huntington's disease. The R.O.S. Activities 101/201 programs and this book are based on the principles and approaches used by the professionals in a skilled setting. This was done for two reasons.

1. Provide family caregivers the basic knowledge and tools to allow them to engage and care for their loved one at home.

2. Offer a starting point that will provide continuity of approach regarding care, communication, and information-gathering to minimize changes and acclimation time if your loved one does have to move from home to an institutional setting.

If you choose to use the services of a home care agency while caring for your loved one at home, please ask if they have a Home Care Certified professional on staff, and verify that the caregiver you choose has received basic training on leisure activities and personal care routines. Has the caregiver been trained on HD? This will assist with continuity of approach, communication, and planning that will benefit both you and your loved one.

Everyone involved in the care for your loved one should be "on the same page" to

minimize changes and challenges that
you and your loved one will face.

Not all family members or friends may
understand or accept your loved one's
disease. This can create conflict. If it helps to
avoid a conflict or stress, please have the
family members read this book or some other
resource prior to a visit so they can begin to
understand the monumental task that you
face as a caregiver. Use visits and interactions
as teaching moments.

It is critical to have as many family members
and friends involved in your loved one's life as
possible. Not just to show your loved one they
are cared for and loved, but also to give you,
the primary family caregiver, the occasional
and much-needed break.

Being a primary caregiver is a 24/7 job.
Without help, you are always on call and
run the risk of becoming physically and
mentally exhausted.

When you do bring in help, make sure all of your loved one's caregivers (full-time, part-time, family, and friends) use the same approach for activities and interaction that you do. With a common approach, there are significantly less opportunities to disrupt routines and make unsettling changes that affect you and your loved one long after the help has left.

A common approach by all is key. Demand it!

The Four Pillars of Activities

There are four areas that you should focus on for engaging your loved one in any type of activity. We call them the Four Pillars of Activities.

First Pillar of Activities: Know your Loved One—Information Gathering and Assessment

Have a Personal History Form completed. Know them—who they are, who they were, and what their functional abilities are today. Make sure all caregivers know this as well.

Second Pillar of Activities: Communicating and Motivating for Success

Communication is key. Each caregiver must know how to effectively communicate with your loved one and be consistent with techniques.

Third Pillar of Activities: Customary Routines and Preferences

As best as possible, maintain a routine and daily plan based on your loved one's needs and preferences.

Fourth Pillar of Activities: Planning and Executing Activities

Based on all of the information you have gathered about your loved one, you have the opportunity to offer engaging activities that are appropriate and meet your loved one's personal preferences.

The Benefits of Activities with a Standard Approach

Caregiver Benefits of Standard Approach to Activities

Planned and well-executed activities result in less stress for you, the caregiver, as well as your loved one. Whether the activity involves playing a game or bathing, a standard approach where as many details as possible are pre-planned can make a significant, positive difference for everyone.

Social Benefits of Activities

Activities offer the opportunity for increased social interaction between family members, friends, caregivers, and the one being cared for. Activities create positive experiences and memories for everyone.

Behavioral Benefits of Activities

Well-planned and well-executed activities of any type can reduce challenging behaviors that sometimes arise when caring for someone.

Self-Esteem Benefits of Activities

Leisure activities offered at the right skill level provide your loved one with an opportunity for success. This is also true with activities of daily living such as dressing. Success during activities improves your loved one's sense of self-esteem.

Sleep Benefits of Activities

When regularly incorporated into a daily routine, activities can improve sleeping at night. If a loved one is inactive all day, it is likely they will nap periodically. Napping can interrupt good sleep patterns at night.

Chapter 3

First Pillar of Activities:
Know Your Loved One—
Information Gathering
and Assessment

For daily caregiving, the first area we need to look at is knowing your loved one. This is the First Pillar of Activities. Knowing your loved one's individual needs, interests, functional abilities, and capacities will assist you in knowing how to plan and provide the care your loved one needs. Please remember when looking at interests—we are talking about interests from your loved one's whole life. You may have all of the information needed after filling out the R.O.S. Personal History Form, but just in case, let's look at the basic information you need to gather.

Name

This is important because how each caregiver addresses your loved one will have a different meaning. For example, your husband's name is Roger Owen Silknitter, and his family and friends called him "Roger the Dodger" or "Dodge."

- Example 1—If you address your husband as "Dodge," he may not recognize you, but he knows he must know you because you know his nickname, so you must be close to him somehow.

- Example 2—When your husband got into trouble at home or school, the authority figure, parent or teacher, called him by his proper name—Roger Owen Silknitter. So if you are trying to get his attention to do things like take medicine, eat, correct a behavior, or move away from an unsafe situation, you may say, "Roger Owen Silknitter, I need you to ..."

- Example 3—At work or with strangers, your husband was known as "Mr. Silknitter." If a caregiver of any type initially addresses him as Mr. Silknitter, he may put up a barrier because he does not recognize them and because he knows from the name used, they do not know him.

Age

What age does your loved one they think they are? This may change as the Huntington's disease progresses. Knowing their personal history will give you clues to what age they think they are which will allow you to better communicate.

Marital Status

Even though your loved one may currently be single, they may have been married or had a significant other in the past. Some people choose to say they are single as opposed to divorced or widowed.

Family Members

Names, relationships, and how close each person has been to your loved one are important.

Religious Preference

Did your loved one go to religious services every week? Any specific requests, communion, or holiday services?

Other Preferences and Habits

Smoking, drinking, favorite foods, sports, knitting, playing cards?

Educational Level

Where did your loved one go to school? What was the mascot? Did they participate in sports or other school activities?

Work Experience

In our adult life, work typically occupies at least 50% of our time. It is important to know what your loved one did, their employer's names, or any significant items that stand out from their career. Here are two examples of why this is important:

- Example 1—It can give you a clue as to what age they think they are and why they might be intent on getting dressed on a particular morning. They may wake up one morning and tell you it is time to go to work and try to leave even though they retired 10 years ago.

- Example 2—Because your loved one spent so much time working throughout their life, their occupation is a treasure trove of topics that you can use in general conversation.

Capabilities

What is your loved one capable of doing for themselves?

This may vary greatly from what they could do prior to the onset of Huntington's disease and can change almost daily.

Caregivers

Who is your loved one the most comfortable with when needing care?

Are they female/male, or a specific caregiver?

Illnesses and Limitations

What other physical illness or limitations does your loved one have? These are as important to know as the personal history information because it allows all caregivers to provide the highest level of care.

As you can see from these examples, details matter. Gather as much information as you can for yourself and all caregivers who may help with your loved one.

Basic knowledge about your loved one is essential. The little things do matter.

There are two important items that you should take note of.

First, any form (like the R.O.S. Personal History Form) that is used to gather personal history should be a living document. It needs constant updating as the Huntington's disease progresses. It is also important to remember that with HD, what works today may not work tomorrow, and it may not work five minutes from now!

Second, you and your loved one may have been very private people. Having Huntington's disease will change that. Gathering information and sharing with other caregivers is critical as your loved one's past pleasures, likes, and activities will become cornerstones of the communication process for everyone.

If there is something that happened years ago that you consider embarrassing or private, and you choose not to share the information, please note that one way or another, it will come out.

Whatever it was that you think is difficult to share, caregivers and family members that offer assistance are not there to judge you or your loved one on something that happened years or even decades ago. They are there to help you in your current moment of need. Information is vital to the communication process and allows all caregivers the opportunity to turn a "bad" day into a "good" day through proper communication techniques.

Your ability to identify past preferences is vital to the planning and execution of an activity. Details matter. Let's look at an example of what we mean.

During their assessments, four people might all say they like "Arts & Crafts," yet they might not actually have the same activity in mind.

- Person 1—Enjoys woodworking and putting together kits (birdhouses, model cars, model airplanes).

- Person 2—Enjoys beading and making jewelry.

- Person 3—Enjoys canvas painting, painting still life objects, or free-form painting.

- Person 4—Enjoys making wreaths for the holidays and changing seasons.

As you can see from these examples, details matter. Gather as much information as you can for yourself and all caregivers who may help with your loved one.

Utilizing the R.O.S. Personal History Form at the back of this book is a starting point to gather as much information as possible. You also may download a copy of the Personal History Form at www.StartSomeJoy.com.

Functional Levels

In addition to the R.O.S. Personal History Form, you also need to look at your loved one's functional level. When planning meaningful activities based on individual interests, you need to also consider your loved one's functional abilities. You need to set them up for success based on what they are able to accomplish. There are several definitions of functional levels. For the purposes of this topic, we will address the following four functioning levels:

Level 1

Your loved one has good social skills. They are able to communicate. They are alert and oriented to person, place, and time, and they have a long attention span.

Level 2

Your loved one has less social skills and their verbal skills may also be impaired. Your loved one may have some behavior symptoms. They may need something to do, and may have an increased energy level, but they have a shorter attention span.

Level 3

Your loved one has less social skills. Their verbal skills are even more impaired than they were at Level 2. They are also easily distracted. Your loved one may have some visual/spatial perception and balance concerns, and they need maximum assistance with their care.

Level 4

Your loved one has a low energy level, nonverbal communication skills, and they rarely initiate contact with others, however, they may respond if given time and cues.

With the personal history and functional level information, you and every caregiver have the greatest opportunity to provide person-appropriate activities for your loved one.

Chapter 4

Second Pillar of Activities: Communicating and Motivating for Success

Communicating and motivating is the Second Pillar of Activities.

Communication is an interactive process where information is exchanged. The ability to respond appropriately, to give feedback on something that was communicated, is just as important as having good listening skills.

Communication with your loved one can be a significant challenge with Huntington's disease. For your loved one, it may be as simple as not being able to find the "right" word to describe something or not finding the words to use or the ability to speak at all.

Talking, reading a book, singing—these are all forms of communication you can utilize.

As the disease progresses, you, your loved one, and all caregivers will have to use various strategies to communicate.

This is due to the many deficits, most particularly cognitive deficits, your loved one will experience. They might end up relying heavily on external cues and guidance from you or other caregivers to achieve some form of effective communication.

The key to effective communication is the ability to listen attentively. That means listening with your ears and eyes and using the knowledge of your loved one's history and habits.

You and all caregivers must make sure that you are listening to your loved one. If their speech slows or they are having difficulty finding the right words, make sure that you give them ample time to try.

Listening goes both ways. Make sure your loved one has heard and understood what you have said. Listening and attention span is decreased in Huntington's disease—just because someone nods their head does not mean that they heard or understood you.

Basic Ideas for You to Use When Communicating with Your Loved One

- Make sure you have your loved one's attention.
- Make eye contact before speaking.
- Rephrase a sentence if needed.
- Speak louder if necessary, but do not yell.
- Use gestures.
- Keep questions and statements simple.
- Ask one question at a time and repeat as needed.
- Pay attention to gestures and facial expressions/changes.

- Allow enough time for your loved one to convey their message.

- Be patient with your loved one.

- Refocus your loved one on the topic if needed.

- Make sure that the message you were trying to convey, no matter what it is, was heard by your loved one.

- When speaking with other caregivers or family members about your loved one in their presence, make sure the conversation is respectful of your loved one. They may move or speak slowly, but assume that they hear everything.

- Be sure to indicate the end of a conversation.

Basic Ideas for How You Can Help Your Loved One

- Encourage them to speak slowly.

- Encourage them to say one word at a time.

- Ask them to repeat the word or sentence when necessary.

- Ask them to rephrase the sentence if needed.

- Describe what your loved one is trying to say, especially if they can't think of the word or indicate the first letter of the word.

- Ask them to speak louder if necessary.

- Encourage them to take a deep breath before speaking. This is helpful if your loved one has some problems breathing.

- Empower them by using alternative techniques, such as word boards, alphabet boards, picture boards, or electronic devices if movement and muscular degeneration are minimal.

- If you do not understand what your loved one said, don't pretend that you do—ask for clarification or repeat what you think was said in the form of a question, such as, "Did you say ...?"

Nonverbal Communication

Although it may seem that most communication happens verbally, research has shown that most communication occurs nonverbally. Nonverbal communication occurs through an individual's body language. There are five key elements to consider in nonverbal communication:

Facial Expressions

Be aware of what your facial expressions are conveying to your loved one. Your mood will be mirrored.

Eye Contact

Ensure that you have made eye contact with your loved one and that their attention is focused on you and what you are saying.

Gestures and Touch

Calmly use nonverbal signs such as pointing, waving, and other hand gestures, in combination with your words.

Tone of Voice

The inflection in your voice helps your loved one relate to the words you are saying.

Body Language

Be aware of the position of your hands and arms when talking to your loved one.

Nonverbal Communication Tips

- Always approach your loved one from the front before speaking to them.

- Smile and extend your hand as to shake their hand. Use touch where welcomed.

- Be at eye level with the person you are talking to.

- Use nonverbal gestures along with words.

- Give nonverbal praises such as smiles and head nods.

- Be an active listener.

- Make sure that all caregivers give your loved one the opportunity and time to speak.

Approaches to Successful Communication and Activities

Be Calm

Always approach your loved one in a relaxed and calm demeanor. Remember, your mood will be mirrored by your loved one. Smiles are contagious.

Be Flexible

There is no right or wrong way of completing a task. Offer praise and encouragement for the effort your loved one puts into a task. If you see your loved one becoming overwhelmed or frustrated, stop the task, and re-approach at another time.

Be Nonresistive

Don't force tasks on your loved one. Adults do not want to be told, "No!" or told what to do. The power of suggestion goes a long way, and you get more with an ounce of sugar than you do a pound of vinegar.

Be Guiding, but Not Controlling

Always use a soft, gentle approach, and remember your tone of voice. Your facial expressions must match the words you are saying.

Barriers to Good Communication

There are generally two barriers that negatively affect communication with your loved one. Here are some tips on how to eliminate negative barriers.

Caregiver Barriers

- Slow down when speaking. Use a calm tone of voice, and be aware of your hand movements.
- Never be demanding or commanding.
- Never argue with a person with impaired cognition. You will never win the argument.
- Enter their world. Live their truth.
- Do not offer long explanations when answering questions.

Environmental Barriers

- Minimize noise from air conditioners and home appliances.

- Turn off the TV if it is on in the same room where you are trying to talk.

- Be aware of outside traffic.

- Check your loved one's hearing aid battery, and make sure that it is not whistling.

- Adjust the lighting in the room. If the lighting in a room makes seeing even more difficult for someone with limited vision, they may be more focused on trying to see rather than on communicating with you.

Validation

In 1963 after years of working with oriented, healthy elderly in community centers, Naomi Feil, the developer of the Validation Therapy techniques, began working with people over the age of 80 who were disoriented. Her initial goals were to help these people face reality and relate to each other in a group. In 1966, she concluded that helping them to face reality is unrealistic. Each person was trapped in a world of fantasy. Exploring feelings and reminiscing encouraged group members to respond better to each. Music stimulated group cohesion and feelings of well-being. Mrs. Feil said, "I abandoned the goal of reality orientation when I found group members withdrew, or became increasingly hostile, whenever I tried to orient them to an intolerable present reality."

To validate is to acknowledge the feelings of a person. To validate is to say that their feelings are true. Denying feelings invalidates the individual. Validation uses empathy to tune into the inner reality of the disoriented old-old. Empathy, or walking in the shoes of the other, builds trust. Trust brings safety. Safety brings strength. Strength renews feelings of worth. Worth reduces stress. With empathy, the Validation worker picks up their clues and helps put their feelings into words. This validates them and restores dignity.

The goals of Validation are:

- Restore self-worth.
- Reduce stress.
- Justify living.
- Work towards resolving unfinished conflicts from the past.
- Reduce the need for chemical and physical restraints.
- Increase verbal and nonverbal communication.
- Prevent withdrawal inward to vegetation.
- Improve gait and physical well-being.

Mrs. Feil is a pioneer, and R.O.S. encourages every caregiver to use Validation instead of reality orientation. Here is an example:

Mr. Smith is frustrated and becoming angry because he can't find his truck keys. Mr. Smith hasn't had his truck in over a year due to his inability to drive. His truck was sold by the family, and he has forgotten that he no longer owns it. Using Validation to ease the distress—the caregiver hands over her personal car keys to Mr. Smith and says, "Here they are." Mr. Smith sets the keys next to him and is relieved that they are no longer lost. When it is time for the caregiver to go, she can take the keys back (likely it won't be a focus any longer since the need was temporarily met). If the caregiver hadn't practiced Validation but instead told Mr. Smith that he can't drive and his family sold his truck, it could have led to distress, anxiety, and increased poor behaviors. In this situation the caregiver would know that Mr. Smith has no intention of getting up and walking away with her keys—he just needed the security of knowing that "His" keys were close by.

Another example: Mr. Smith is sitting at his door waiting for the bus to come and pick him up. He isn't engaging with you the caregiver and isn't willing to participate in an activity, have lunch, or go for a walk because he feels he can't miss the bus. This could be a triggered memory from his past where he rode the bus to and from work and home. The incorrect way to handle this situation is to orient Mr. Smith that there is no bus coming and that he is already home. As in the example above, this could cause unneeded distress, increased confusion, anger, and other behaviors. Using Validation, the caregiver would inform Mr. Smith that the bus is scheduled to be here tomorrow, or the bus broke down and isn't going to be up and running until tomorrow, or the bus won't be here for a couple of hours so let's do this …—and divert his attention to a task at hand. Like many who suffer from some short-term memory loss, the conversation won't be remembered the next day, and the whole situation may be repeated.

Taking extra time with loved ones so they feel comfortable expressing their feelings and concerns is important. As the caregiver, use that time to validate and listen intently to what they are really trying to communicate to you.

As the disease progresses, your loved one may not be able verbalize their needs and concerns. By using Validation through sensory touch programs, music, and one-on-one companionship, their needs can be met. These Validation techniques are also beneficial for bed-bound loved ones. Providing care for nonverbal loved ones and/or bed-bound loved ones utilizing information from the R.O.S. Personal History Form will be crucial to providing the quality care they need.

Communication and Behavior

Behaviors are a means to communicate when words are no longer effective.

Caregivers must uncover the meaning behind the behaviors and put a plan in place to manage those needs. Remember, be a detective. Validation techniques will be successful here also.

Aggressive Behaviors

Aggressive behaviors can be defined as hitting, angry outbursts, using obscenities, yelling, verbalizing racial insults, making inappropriate sexual comments, and/or biting. Trying to communicate with or provide care to a person who is aggressive can be stressful and even frightening for caregivers.

Possible Causes for Aggression

- Too much noise or overstimulation—
  Examples: The television is on, the dogs are barking, and an occupational therapist just walked in the door to begin a session.

- Cluttered environment—
  Example: The house or the room your loved one is in is a mess.

- Uncomfortable room temperatures.

- Basic needs not being met—
Examples: Your loved one may be hungry, thirsty, needing to use the bathroom, or needing comfort.

- Pain of any type—
Examples: Your loved one may have a headache, sore bottom from rash, or diabetic nerve pain.

- Fear, anxiety or confusion—
Examples: Your loved one may be lashing out both verbally and physically, experiencing paranoia, anger, or denial, or they be making accusatory remarks.

- Communication barriers—These barriers can come in many different forms in response to mental and physical impairments. Communication barriers can be a result of depression, physical limitations related to diagnosis, word salad (random words together in a sentence that's nonsensical), or the inability to focus and/or complete a thought to verbalize needs and concerns. Additional communication barriers include:

◦ Fear or anxiety from not recognizing their surroundings—
Example: Your loved one moved in with you two years ago when their health became a concern. They left the only house they had ever lived in during their adult life. Their cognitive deficits are causing them to believe that they are 30 years younger and still live at their old home, and they want to go home.

◦ Caregiver's mood—
Example: They can read you and all caregivers like a book. If you are having a bad day, leave it in the other room or at the door before you walk in to interact with your loved one.

◦ Feeling that they are being rushed—

Examples: Quickly moving from one activity to another, taking dishes off the table or counter before your loved one is finished eating, or asking various times, "Are you finished?" or "Are you done?"

- Difficulty seeing activity or materials used for an activity, which may prevent them from participating—
Example: Visual impairment or cognitive deficits that inhibit participation in activities of preference.

- Lack of independence—
Examples: Needing assistance with personal grooming, needing assistance with daily routines (preparing meals, turning on the TV, going out of the home, dressing, and completing household chores).

The feeling and awareness of the loss of independence can be extremely difficult for your loved one to accept. It is an area to confront with caution, dignity, and grace. It is imperative that caregivers allow their loved ones to do as much as they are able to do independently with physician approval and standby assistance. A great loss of independence at a fast pace can cause negative outcomes for your loved one.

Interventions to Utilize to Mitigate Aggressive Behaviors

- Identify the triggers of the aggression. Be a detective. There is never a behavior that just occurs.

- Communicate for success. Use the skills you have learned in this book. Be guiding, but not controlling.

- Reminisce with your loved one about specific details of their past. This is why knowledge of your loved one and who they were is so important.

- Validate and support their feelings.

- Remain calm, and speak in a soft tone.

- Find items that they find comfort in, e.g., a picture of the family.

- Provide consistent caregivers and schedules. Stick to your loved one's routine.

- Engage in recreational activities that match your loved one's abilities and interests, as tolerated.

- Break down instructions into one-step increments.

- Keep an ongoing dialogue between family members and caregivers over any noted changes in patterns or behaviors.

- Help your loved one to slow down and relax.

- Play or listen to music your loved one enjoys for its calming effects.

- Use spiritual support if this is important to your loved one.

Chapter 5

Third Pillar of Activities:
Customary Routines
and Preferences

The Third Pillar of Activities is the daily routine. For the purpose of developing a daily plan of care, we will be discussing two areas: Daily Customary Routine and Activity Preferences. The goal is to gain from your loved one's perspective how important certain aspects of care and activity are to them as an individual and work those items into their routine.

When caring for your loved one at home, this very well could mean a disruption to your personal daily routine, but that might be a necessary trade off to minimize behavioral issues that might become very wearing on you and your loved one.

Daily Customary Routine

Your loved one has distinct lifestyle preferences, and they should be preserved to the fullest extent possible. All reasonable accommodation should be made to maintain their lifestyle preferences.

Not accommodating your loved one's lifestyle preferences can contribute to depressed mood and increased behavior symptoms. When a person feels like their control has been removed and that their preferences are not respected as an individual, it can be demoralizing.

Let us look at an example of a daily routine and how Huntington's disease may alter that routine in a way that you might not be prepared for, but must adjust for.

You have been caring for your mother, Esther, for several months. You know based on her life history assessment that cooking has always played a major role in her life. Specifically, your mother cooked for you and your brother when you were kids. Your brother, John, happens to live nearby, and he is able to come over for lunch with Mom every day. Recently, the speed of the progression of the disease has accelerated. Because of the rapid progression, prepping, cooking, and cleaning up afterwards, which she likes to do, has become almost impossible.

John has offered to bring in lunch daily to share with Mom but this upsets her as she has always been the provider of meals.

John does begin to bring in take-out daily for lunch. Within a couple of days of this "new routine," Esther begins to display behaviors that are uncharacteristic to her personality. She begins withdrawing from mealtime conversation, asking for assistance with tasks that she was previously doing independently, and showing a lack of motivation for other activities. You begin to notice the decline increasing each week in the absence of cooking. As a detective, you begin to analyze the situation. Working with her doctors, you first discover that medically, nothing has really changed. You then look at items around the house and routines, and you realize that the behaviors started when John started bringing lunch over daily and your mother was not allowed to try cooking. You put a plan in place to see if it is the inability to do something she loves that gives her meaning and purpose, cooking, that is causing the current issues. You contact John and let him know he does not need to bring lunch tomorrow. That evening you ask Esther, "What is your favorite thing to cook for lunch?" You ask even though you already know the answer from her Personal History Form. You ask to get her involved in the process.

In the morning following breakfast, you surprise Esther with all of the ingredients needed to prepare her favorite lunch. You provide a safe and sturdy stool for Esther to sit at the counter and stove area and begin to assist her in putting everything together. You provide hands-on assistance as needed but allow Esther to do the majority of the preparations. After lunch is complete, Esther requests to have the stool moved to the sink so that she can wash the dishes. This routine consumed Esther's morning and most of the afternoon, but you notice that Esther is smiling. Esther is talkative. Esther is engaging with you and her son throughout the process, and the declines that you noted in the weeks prior have all but disappeared on this day. After you've evaluated your cooking experiment, you discuss the modifications you would need to continue to allow Esther to do what she loves with John, e.g., additional stools, large-grip and large-handle utensils and pans, weekly meal planning, and groceries.

Doing the best you can to maintain your loved one's preferences is critical to maintaining quality of life.

Activity Preferences

Activities are a way for individuals to establish meaning in their lives. The *need* for enjoyable activities does not change with age or growing health needs. The only thing that changes is the level of assistance individuals may need in order to engage in those pursuits.

A lack of opportunity to engage in meaningful and enjoyable activities can result in boredom, depression, and behavioral disturbances.

Individuals vary in the activities they prefer, reflecting unique personalities, past interests, religious and cultural background, plus changing physical and mental abilities. We as family caregivers have a great opportunity to empower a loved one to see that they possess many great talents and abilities. By modifying or adapting activities to allow them to engage at an independent level, you are restoring their self-esteem and self-worth.

Chapter 6

Fourth Pillar of Activities: Planning and Executing Activities

Planning and executing is the Fourth Pillar of Activities. With the knowledge of your loved one's history, functional level, effective communication techniques to use, and their daily routine, we now look at planning activities in which they can be successful.

The Lesson Plan

The Lesson Plan template is a guideline for an activity. Each loved one's abilities and responses are different. This will dictate how you modify an activity to meet their individual needs and abilities. The Lesson Plan is an ever-changing document. It is meant to be written on and note any changes that are needed so the next person working with your loved one can follow your modifications in hopes of recreating a positive experience.

Items in the Lesson Plan

Date

Document the date the activity is used.

Activity Name

You can rename the activity if you or your loved one prefers.

Objective of Activity

Our goal is to provide meaningful activities. People have a need to be productive, and they want to engage in something with a purpose. List the objectives of the activity.

Materials

The list of suggested materials to use with this activity.

Prerequisite Skills

The skills your loved one needs to participate in this activity.

Activity Outline

Step-by-step instructions to complete this activity.

Evaluation

When you or a family member are conducting an activity with your loved one, documenting results and responses is critical to improve activity programs for your loved one. Items to document:

- Verbal cues, physical assistance, or modifications you make to activity.

- Your loved one's response to this activity.

- Did your loved one enjoy this activity or not?

- Was the activity successful at distracting or eliminating a negative behavior?

A blank template is included on the next page to give you an example of what a Lesson Plan looks like.

Lesson Plan Blank Example

Date	Activity Name

Objective of Activity

Materials

Prerequisite Skills

Activity Outline

Evaluation

Chapter 7

Leisure Activity
Categories, Types, Topics, and Tips

Activity Categories

Activities are generally broken down into three different categories: Maintenance Activities, Supportive Activities, and Empowering Activities.

Maintenance Activities

Maintenance activities are traditional activities that help your loved one maintain physical, cognitive, social, spiritual, and emotional health. Examples include:

- Religious activities (attending a service, daily devotions, reading scripture)

- Watching TV

- Reading (books, magazines, newspaper)

- Games (puzzles, Sudoku, word finds, crossword puzzles, cards, board games)
- Walking
- Events
- Outings

Supportive Activities

Supportive activities are for those that have a lower tolerance for traditional activities. These types of activities provide a comfortable environment while providing stimulation or solace. Examples include:

- Listening to and singing music
- Hand massages
- Relaxation activities such as aromatherapy, meditation, and bird-watching

Empowering Activities

Empowering activities help your loved one attain self-respect by receiving opportunities

for self-expression and responsibility.
Examples include:

- Cooking
- Making memory boxes
- Folding laundry

Activity Types

Once you have chosen an activity from a category that will suit your loved one's need, you must choose an activity type that will interest them. There are several types of activities to choose from. Below are some examples:

Art Activities

- Coloring
- Painting
- Dancing

Craft Activities

- Jewelry making
- Knitting

- Scrapbooking
- Woodworking
- Model Building

Verbal Activities

- Conversation
- Trivia
- Reminiscing

Entertainment Activities

- Board games
- Card games
- Video games
- Crossword puzzles

Listening Activities

- Music
- Storytelling
- Books on tape
- Memory games
- Listening to the radio

Visual Activities

- Watching a movie
- Watching a performance

Writing Activities

- Writing a story or poem
- Writing a letter
- Writing a life history

Active Activities

- Dancing
- Folding laundry
- Road trips
- Cooking
- Walking

Activity Topics

Once you know what category of activity you want to use to engage your loved one, here are some suggestions for topics the activity can be based on:

Colors

- Colors of their favorite sports team
- Colors of their wedding
- Colors of flowers or cars

Music

- Favorite music
- Music from when they were younger and dating
- Patriotic songs
- Holiday songs
- Favorite artists from the age they think they are, e.g., if they believe they are 25 years old, use popular singers or songs of that era.

Military Service

- War stories
- World events of their time—or time of age they think they are
- Their personal experiences of either military service or what it was like in the States

Holidays

- Specific holidays that coincide with their culture or religion
- Favorite holidays
- Traditions

Cooking

- Home cooking
- Comfort food
- Favorite recipes from their mother or grandmother
- Favorite food associated with events, holidays, family gatherings

Sports

- Professional sports teams they like
- Their involvement in sports
- Big sporting events from their era

School Days

- Where they went to school
- Favorite school classes or teachers
- Memories of their children's school events

Old Cars

- Their family's first car
- Their first car
- Prices of cars now and then
- Dream cars

Places

- Where they were born
- Where they grew up
- Places they have been
- Vacations they took

Activity Tips for Individuals
with Mild to Moderate Cognitive Deficits

Many loved ones have cognitive deficits that are significant enough to impact their day as well as their awareness of their surroundings. By providing activities that reinforce their past, we increase and improve their social skills which can improve their general interactions with others.

Validating Activities

Validating activities validate the memories and feelings of individuals who are much disoriented. They focus on your loved one's perception of what happened in the past.

Reminiscing Activities

Reminiscing activities are designed to help your loved one identify the important contributions he or she has made throughout their lifetime. It is an important part of human development to see oneself as a contributing member of society.

Resocializing Activities

Once your loved one can successfully participate in reminiscing and validating activities, it is time to encourage them, through resocializing activities, to build on social skills and begin to expand their connections to the community in which they live. This can be as simple as connecting with a neighbor, a friend within the church, or a friend within the community.

Chapter 8

Activities of Daily Living
Tips and Suggestions

With Huntington's disease, customary daily living and preferences may change when least expected.

Bathing

Bathing can be a relaxing, enjoyable experience—or a time of confrontation and anger. Use a calm approach. Your loved one's "usual" routine is very important.

Safety and Preparation

- Water temperature should range from 110-115 degrees Fahrenheit maximum to prevent burning or skin injury.

- Hot water can cause fatigue.

- The floor of the tub needs to be slip proof. Use a rubber mat that does not slide, or use permanent nonslip decals.

- Place a nonskid rug on the floor outside the tub to prevent slipping.

- Install grab bars. Always make sure the grab bars are properly and securely installed into the wall studs.

- Do not use bath oils.

Bathing—Know Your Loved One

- Is your loved one accustomed to a bath or shower?

- Can they get into a bath or shower without assistance?

- Can they soap their body or wash their hair independently?

- Can they dry independently with a towel, with simple tricks such as sewing straps onto the towel to make the towel easier to hold?

- If help is needed, who is your loved one the most comfortable with when needing assistance bathing?

- It can be awkward waiting and watching someone perform a task. Instead, you can provide supervision, but be doing something else. For instance, getting towels out while your loved one is undressing is an effective use of the time and space. Or washing your loved one's lower body while they wash their upper body deflects this discomfort. This also creates a sense of support versus a feeling of total dependence.

Bathing—Communicating and Motivating

If you have to help a loved one bathe:

- Allow your loved one to do what is within their control.

- Stay friendly and respectful.

- Try to avoid arguments by offering a combination of visual cues, step-by-step setup, and short verbal cues.

Bathing—Customary Routines and Preferences

- What time of day does our loved one normally bathe?

- How often did your loved one bathe before the onset of Huntington's disease?

- What is the process that works for you and your loved one when it is time to bathe? Make sure all caregivers know each detail of the process. For example:

  ○ Is the water turned on and running prior to your loved one entering the tub?

  ○ Is a towel placed on a shower chair seat so that that your loved one may avoid a chill on their bottom when seated in the shower?

- Whatever the process, take it one step at a time, following your loved one's normal bathing routine. For example, your loved one may prefer that you wash their hair first and then their body—or they may prefer to soak for 10 minutes before washing.

- When assisting your loved one to bathe, have a towel ready to put over the shoulders or on the lap to minimize feelings of exposure.

Bathing—Planning and Executing

- Have all care items and tools ready prior to starting the bath process.

  ○ A shower chair if necessary.

  ○ A handheld hose for showering and bathing.

  ○ A long-handled sponge or scrubbing brush if self scrubbing is desired.

- Sponges with soap inside or a soft soap applicator instead of bar soap (bar soap can easily slip out of your loved one's hand).

- Have a towel and clothing prepared for when the bath is finished.

- A second towel can be placed on the back of a chair to allow your loved one to dry their back by rubbing on the towel or you might use a terry cloth robe instead of a towel for drying.

Other Bathroom & Grooming Activities

Brushing Teeth

- Start with step-by-step directions. This may not be as simple as you might think. Take a moment and think of all of the steps necessary to brush your teeth, from walking into the bathroom, to finding the toothpaste in the drawer and removing the cap, to rinsing your mouth once you have finished brushing. Depending on your loved one's level of cognitive change, it might be easier to show them.

- For family members at home, brush your teeth at the same time as your loved one.

- Use positive reinforcement and compliment your loved one on the good job they are doing.

- Help your loved one to clean their dentures as needed.

Shaving

- Encourage a male to shave.
- Use an electric razor for safety.
- If they need assistance, please provide it.
- Give positive feedback, and do not verbally correct.

Makeup

- If your loved one had been accustomed to wearing makeup prior to the onset of Huntington's disease, there is no reason for this to stop. If she shows interest or desire to wear makeup, encourage her to do so, and offer assistance to apply if needed.

Hair

- Try to maintain hairstyle and care as your loved one did.

- Explain each step in simple terms before you do anything to reduce any anxiety.

Nails

- Keep nails clean and trimmed. Be gentle while trimming your loved one's nails. Be mindful of how you pull and where you place their fingers and arms.

- If your loved one had a regular schedule for nail care prior to the onset of Huntington's disease or other health issues, please try to maintain that schedule.

- Offer to polish your loved one's nails.

- When polishing, engage your loved one in conversation.

Toileting or Using the Bathroom

- Learn your loved one's individual's habits and routines for using the toilet. This may not be something that you knew before and is part of the changing roles.

- Toilet routinely on rising, before and after meals, and at bedtime, at a minimum.

- If your loved one is having trouble communicating, please watch for agitation, pulling at their clothes, or restlessness. This may be an indication of a need to go to the bathroom.

- Assist with clothing as needed, and be positive and pleasant while assisting.

- Provide verbal cues and instructions as needed. Be guiding, but not controlling.

Clothing

Clothing—Know Your Loved One

- Daily clothing choices should remain as they had been before the onset of Huntington's disease and based on their available wardrobe during the initial stages of the disease.

- As their Huntington's disease progresses, changes will have to be made. Clothes need to be comfortable and easy to remove, especially to go to bathroom.

- Choose clothes that are loose fitting and have elastic waistbands.

- For convenience, choose wraparound clothing instead of the pullover type.

- If possible, choose clothing that opens in the front, not the back. This prevents your loved one from having to reach behind their body and allows the feeling of independence from dressing oneself.

- When purchasing new clothes, look for clothing with large, flat buttons; Velcro closures, or zippers.

- To assist your loved one with zipping pants or a jacket, attach a zipper pull or leather loop on the end of the zipper.

- Choose slip-on shoes.

Clothing—Communicating and Motivating

- Use short, simple sentences.
- Provide verbal cues and instructions as needed.
- Always smile.
- Talk calmly and gently.
- Do not argue, or try to explain "why."

Clothing—Routines and Preferences

- Have a friendly discussion each evening about the next day's schedule and what your loved one may want to wear.

- For individuals with Huntington's disease, changes will have to be made as any cognitive deficits progress. You may have to limit the choice of clothing, and leave only two outfit options in their room at a time.

- If your loved one wants to wear the same thing every day, and if you can afford it, buy three or four sets of the same clothing.

Clothing—Planning and Executing

- Clothes should be laid out according to what goes on first.

- Avoid clothes that are most difficult for your loved one—such as panty hose, knee-high nylons, tight socks, or high heels.

- Make sure that items are not inside out and that buttons, zips, and fasteners are all undone before handing the clothes to your loved one.

Dressing

Dressing—Know Your Loved One

Initially, your loved one may just need verbal cues and instructions on dressing. Please remember to allow them to dress independently as long as possible to foster an ongoing sense of dignity and independence. As the primary caregiver, you will have to be the judge as to when all caregivers need to begin assisting your loved one with dressing.

Dressing—Communicating and Motivating

- Use short, simple sentences. Provide verbal cues and instructions as needed.

- If your loved one is confused, give instructions in very short steps, such as, "Now put your arm through the sleeve." It may help to use actions to demonstrate these instructions.

- Give praise as justified as each step is accomplished.

86

- Always smile.

- Speak calmly and gently.

- Do not argue, or try to explain "why."

- Remember to ask your loved one if they would like to go to the toilet before getting dressed.

Dressing—Routines and Preferences

- Does your loved one get dressed first thing in the morning—before or after breakfast?

- Does your loved one change into pajamas right before bed or after dinner?

- Try to maintain your loved one's preferred routine for as long as possible.

- Little things matter. For example, your loved one may like to put on all underwear before putting on anything else. Know their preferences.

Dressing—Planning and Executing

- Think about privacy. Make sure that blinds or curtains are closed and that no one will walk in and disturb your loved one while they are dressing.

- Make sure the room is warm enough to get dressed in.

- Hand your loved one a single item at a time.

- To assist with balance, let your loved one get dressed while sitting in a chair that has armrests.

- If it is of help, have your loved one use a dressing stick to get a coat or shirt on or off.

- If putting on pants independently, have your loved one roll from side to side to get pants over hips. This can be done while sitting in a chair or lying down on a bed.

- If needed, have your loved one use a button hook to button clothing.

If mistakes are made—for example, by putting something on the wrong way—be tactful, or find a way for you both to laugh about it.

***Note**: Wearing several layers of thin clothing rather than one thick layer can be helpful. With layers, your loved one will be able to remove a layer if too warm.

Remember that your loved one may get to a point where they are no longer able to tell you if they are too hot or cold, so keep an eye out for signs of discomfort.

Eating

Eating—Know Your Loved One

- Keep long-standing personal preferences in mind when preparing food. However, be aware that your loved one may suddenly develop new food preferences or reject foods that they enjoyed in the past.

89

- Can your loved one eat independently?

- Does your loved one have a visual impairment that may affect their ability to see a meal or drink? Due to normal changes in our eyesight as we age, eating and dining may offer additional challenges.

Meals—Communicating and Motivating

- Use short, simple sentences.

- Provide verbal cues and instructions as needed.

- Give your loved one your full attention.

- Always smile, talk calmly and gently.

- Be guiding, but not controlling.

Meals—Routines and Preferences

- No matter what time of day breakfast, lunch, and dinner are served, be consistent every day.

- Offer snacks throughout the day.

- Limit distractions. Serve meals in quiet surroundings, away from the television and other activities.

- Factor into the overall schedule of the day that each meal or snack may take an hour or longer to finish eating.

Meals—Planning and Executing

This is a particular area to pay attention to during meals. Below are tips covering several areas to help you with your loved one:

Appropriate Lighting, Glare and Contrast

- Reduce glare by having your loved one sit with the sunlight behind them when eating.

- Use lighting which illuminates the entire dining space and makes objects visible, as well as reducing shadows or reflections.

Creating Clear Visual Distinctions

- Use solid colors with no distracting patterns.

- When pouring a light-colored drink, such as milk, use a dark glass.

- When pouring a dark-colored drink, such as cola, use a white glass.

- Avoid clear glasses. They can disappear from view.

- Use white dishes when eating dark-colored food, and use dark dishes when eating light-colored food.

- To make dishes easier to find on the table, use a tablecloth or placemats that are the opposite color of the dishes.

*Note: Fiesta ware colors (yellow/tangerine) contrast with most foods so they can be easily seen and will enhance visual perception.

Setting the Table

- Have your loved one help in the kitchen and set the table if they are able.

- Set the table for every meal as your loved one is used to.

- Use a non-skid mat for objects placed on the table.

- Use a plate with a raised lip to prevent food from spilling.

- Use utensils with lightweight, built-up handles.

- Use a long straw with a no-spill cup, or use a plastic mug with a large handle.

If you are new to caregiving for this particular loved one and they are unable to help or tell you how they set the table, please:

- Set each place setting in the same way for every meal.

- Place the knife and spoon to the right of the plate.

- Place the fork and napkin to the left of the plate.

- Place the glass or cup above the plate to the right or left, depending on whether your loved one is left- or right-handed.

- Decide how to set the rest of the table—main dish, side dishes, seasonings, and condiments. Do it the same way each day.

Other Meal Considerations

- Your loved one may not be able to tell if something is too hot to eat or drink. Always test the temperature of foods and beverages before serving.

- Make meals an enjoyable social event so everyone looks forward to the experience.

- Clean up spills immediately.

- Let your loved one know it is okay to rest their elbows on the table to provide more motion at the wrist and hand.

Meals and Cognitive Deficits

Eating a meal can be a challenge for your loved one with Huntington's disease. Here are some simple techniques that can help reduce mealtime problems:

Meal Preparation for Early-Stage Huntington's Disease

If your loved one wants to assist in making a meal:

- Make sure your cabinets are organized with each item labeled with large easy-to-see labels.

- Use simple written or verbal step-by-step instructions.

- You or another caregiver must perform tasks using sharp objects, such as knives, and assume operation of the stove or oven.

- When using a stove top, use the back burners, and turn the handles inward toward the back of the stove to avoid any potential grabbing of the pots or pans.

If you are not there to supervise because you have to go to work:

- Avoid planning meals that require use of the stove. Your loved one may not remember to turn off the stove and may not be able to distinguish between a pot that is hot or cold.

- Lay out the ingredients of a meal on the counter or in the refrigerator in labeled containers in the order that your loved one will use them—similar to laying out their clothes at night.

- Transfer bulk items, including milk, from a larger container to a smaller container that will be easier to lift and pour.

Meal Preparation for Higher-Level Huntington's Disease

- Try to have all meals eaten at a kitchen or dining table or a chair with a serving tray.

- Avoid meals in bed, if possible—let the bed be for sleeping.

Activities of daily living can be challenging, but they can be accomplished. Making sure that all caregivers know your loved one, their routine, and the game plan for any activity, will help you and your loved one be successful.

Chapter 9

Put Your Mask on First

There will be many challenges to you personally in this caregiving journey that can and will wear you down. As a caregiver, first and foremost, you must take care of yourself in order to be able to assist your loved one. That might be easier said than done, but please make every effort to do so. The following are some general tips for you, the family caregiver:

About You

- Put yourself first (this is not being selfish)—if you are not in good physical or mental health you cannot help anyone.

- Arrange some time for yourself.

- Keep a strong support system.

- Do not be afraid to ask for help.

- Keep contact with friends.

- Define priorities; do not try to be all things to all people.

Stress

- Recognize your own stress and take steps to minimize. Stress can be exhibited in multiple ways:
  - Anger
  - Helplessness
  - Embarrassment
  - Grief
  - Depression
  - Isolation
  - Physical illness

Burnout

Burnout for caregivers results from physical and emotional exhaustion.

It is important to realize a family member, spouse or hired caregiver experiences the same emotions as staff in health care facilities, but may not have the needed support system. Suggestions to avoid burnout:

- Know what makes you angry or impatient. Make a list.

- Look for the reason behind behavior.

- Use relaxation techniques, e.g., deep breathing, imagery, and music.

- Ask for help, and accept help when it is offered!

Caregiving is a challenging road with constant twists and turns, from the change in your role/relationship with your loved one, to dealing with the strains of a 24/7 job of caring for that loved one. As much as you may feel like you are alone, please know that you are not. Millions of family caregivers are dealing with the same issues that you are. Do not be embarrassed to share details about what you are experiencing, and do not be afraid to ask for help. There are individuals, organizations, and support groups throughout the country that are available to you. There is also R.O.S. —we were built on the simple mission of our founder's need to help his mother and father during a 25-year battle with Parkinson's and dementia. We understand what you are going through, and we are here to help.

Personal History Form

This is _____'s Personal History

Name: _____

Maiden Name: _____

Date of Birth: _____

Preferred Name: _____

Name and relationship of people completing this history:

_____

_____

_____

What age do you think the person thinks they are?

_____

Do they ask for their spouse/partner but do not recognize them?

_____

Do they look for their children but do not recognize them?

_____

Do they look for their mom? _____

Do they perceive themselves as younger? Please describe.

_____

_____

Describe the "home" they remember. _____

_____

_____

_____

Describe the person's personality prior to the onset of
Huntington's disease. _____

_____

_____

What makes the person feel valued? Talents, occupation,
accomplishments, family, etc. _____

_____

_____

What are some favorite items they must always have in
sight or close by? _____

_____

_____

What is their exact morning routine?

_____

_____

_____

_____

What is their exact evening routine?

_____

_____

_____

_____

What type of clothing do they prefer? Do they like to choose their own clothes for the day, or do they prefer to have their clothes laid out for them?

_____

_____

_____

_____

What is their favorite beverage?

_____

What is their favorite food?

_____

What will get them motivated? (Church, friends coming over, going out, etc.)

_____

_____

_____

_____

List significant interests in their life, such as hobbies, recreational activities, job related skills/experiences, military experience, etc.

- Age 8 to 20:

_____

_____

_____

- Age 20 to 40:

_____

_____

_____

What is their religious background? (Affiliation, prayer time, symbols, traditions, church/synagogue name, etc. Did they lead any services or sing in the choir?)

_____

_____

_____

What type of music do they enjoy listening to, playing, or singing? Do they have any musical talents?

_____

_____

_____

What is their favorite TV program? Movie?

_____

_____

_____

Did they enjoy reading? Which authors, topics, or genres do they prefer? Would they listen to audiobooks or books on tape?

_____

_____

_____

_____

Can they tell the difference between someone on TV and a real person?

_____

_____

Include names of spouses/partners, dates of marriage, and other relevant information. (If married more than once, provide specifics for each partner.)

_____

_____

_____

_____

_____

List distinct characteristics about his/her spouse/partner(s), such as occupations, personality traits, or daily routine.

_____

_____

_____

_____

_____

Do they have children? Be sure to include children both living and deceased. Include names, birth dates, and any other relevant information.

_____

_____

_____

_____

_____

Who do they ask for the most? What is their relationship with this person(s)? Describe how that person typically spends their day.

_____

_____

_____

_____

_____

What causes your loved one stress?

_____

_____

_____

_____

**What calms them down when they are stressed
or agitated?**

_____

_____

_____

_____

**Other information that would help bring joy to
your loved one.**

_____

_____

_____

_____

_____

_____

_____

_____

_____

About the Authors

Scott Silknitter

Scott Silknitter is the founder of R.O.S. Therapy Systems. He designed and created the R.O.S. Play Therapy™ System, the *How Much Do You Know About* Series of themed activity books, and the R.O.S. *BIG Book*. Starting with a simple backyard project to help Mom and Dad, Mr. Silknitter has dedicated his life to improving the quality of life for all seniors through meaningful education, entertainment and activities.

Robert D. Brennan, RN, NHA, MS, CDP

Robert Brennan is a Registered Nurse and Nursing Home Administrator with over 35 years of experience in long-term care. He is a Certified Dementia Practitioner and is Credentialed in Montessori-Based Dementia Programming (MBDP) providing general and Train the Trainer programs. Robert was responsible for the development of an Assisted Living Federation of America (ALFA) "Best of the Best" award-winning program for care of individuals with dementia using MBDP. He currently provides education on dementia and long-term regulatory topics.

Vanessa Emm, BA, ACC/EDU, AC-BC, CDP

Vanessa Emm is a Certified Activity Consultant/ Instructor/Educator through the National Certification Council of Activity Professionals (NCCAP), a Consultant through the National Association of Activity Professionals Credentialing Center (NAAPCC), and a Certified Dementia Practitioner through the National Council of Certified Dementia Practitioners (NCCDP). Vanessa currently serves as the Operations Trustee for the National Association of Activity Professionals (NAAP). Vanessa has been in the long-term care field for the past 12 years. She currently works as an Activity Consultant (TaggEmm Consulting), Public Relations/Marketing Director for South Lyon Medical Center and provides educational/consultant services to facilities throughout Northern Nevada. She has presented at national conferences, state conferences and workshops. Vanessa received her Bachelor's Degree in Gerontology from Minnesota State University Moorhead with an emphasis in Biology and additional training in research and grant writing.

References

1. *The Handbook of Theories on Aging* (Bengtson et al., 2009)
2. *Activity Keeps Me Going & Going, Volume 1*, (Peckham et al., 2011)
3. *Essentials for the Activity Professional in Long-Term Care* (Lanza, 1997)
4. *Abnormal Psychology*, Butcher
5. www.dhspecialservices. com
6. National Certification Council for Dementia Practitioners, www.NCCDP.org
7. "Managing Difficult Dementia Behaviors: An A-B-C Approach" By Carrie Steckl
8. Iowa Geriatric Education Center website, Marianne Smith, PhD, ARNP, BC Assistant Professor University of Iowa College of Nursing
9. *Excerpts taken from "Behavior...Whose Problem is it?" Hommel, 2012
10. *Merriam-Webster's Dictionary*
11. "The Latent Kin Matrix" (Riley, 1983)
12. *Care Planning Cookbook* (Nolta et al. 2007)
13. "Long-Term Care" (Blasko et al. 2011)
14. "Success-Oriented Programs for the Dementia Client" (Worsley et al 2005)
15. Heerema, Esther. "Eight Reasons Why Meaningful Activities Are Important for People with Dementia." www.about.com
16. *Validation: The Feil Method* (Feil, 1992)
17. *Activities 101 for the Family Caregiver* (Appler-Worsley, Bradshaw, Silknitter)
18. www.hda.org.
19. American Foundation for the Blind
20. www.aging.com
21. www.WebMD.com
22. www.caregiver.org

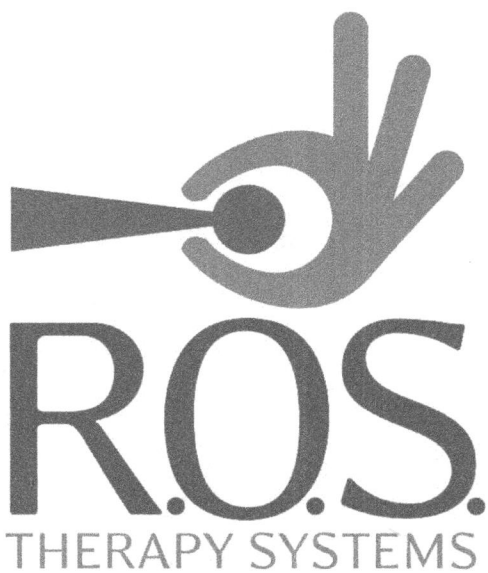

R.O.S.

THERAPY SYSTEMS

For additional assistance, please contact us at:
www.ROSTherapySystems.com
888-352-9788